Index

1

What Is Tube Feeding?

Some people may not be able to eat, drink, or swallow. If they cannot eat enough or even at all, they will receive nutrition through a feeding tube.

Everyone needs nutrition for daily life and you may have increased nutrient needs if you're recovering from a recent injury, surgery, or other condition. Your body needs the basic building blocks of nutrition to restore or maintain good health. These components include protein, carbohydrates, fat, vitamins, minerals, and water. All of these nutrients work together to provide you energy and nutrients which will help your body to work as well as it can.

Tube feeding can be long or short term. If you need tube feeding when you're discharged from the hospital, you will have a gastrostomy tube (PEG), Jejunosotomy (J-tube) or transgastric jejunostomy (PEG-J) tube placed to provide nutrition. These tubes bypass your mouth and esophagus. They are inserted into your stomach or intestine through a hole in the abdominal wall. You can use the tube for nutrition, hydration, and medications.

Tube Types

When you have a tube placed for enteral nutrition, your physician will place one of three types of tubes: gastrostomy, gastrojejunal, or jejunostomy. Each tube is designed for a specific purpose and your physician or dietitian can explain the reason for your tube type.

- **Gastrostomy Tubes**

A gastrostomy tube, also frequently referred to as a PEG (percutaneous endoscopic gastrostomy) is the most common type of tube. A tube will pass from your abdominal wall to your stomach and be anchored with a balloon or bolster to keep it in place. This type of tube may be used for bolus, gravity, or pump assisted tube feeds.

- **Gastrojejunal Tubes**

This type of tube can be recommended if you have a problem with stomach emptying, pancreatitis, or other conditions. With this tube, the procedure will pass a tube through your stomach but the tube will end in the first part of your small intestine, the jejunum, instead of the stomach. With a gastrojejunal tube (GJ-tube), you will need to have pump-assisted tube feeds.

- **Jejunostomy Tubes**

This type of tube may be recommended if you have stomach damage, partial or total stomach removal, or other problems that would make it impossible to place a gastrostomy tube. The procedure involves inserting a tube from the abdominal wall into the first section of the small intestine known as the jejunum. With this type of tube, you will need to have pump-assisted feeds

You have a ____

Tube Feeding Supplies

When you go home with tube feeding, you'll need specific supplies to manage your tube feeds at home. Your home care agency may provide some of these supplies or you may need to purchase them. Your healthcare team will fill in the bubbles for the supplies you need.

- o Tube Feeding Formula
- o 60 mL Syringe
- o Tube Feed Adaptor
- o Tube Feed Pump
- o Tube Feed Pump Set- Bag/Container and Tubing

Tube Feeding Formulas

With tube feeding, you will be given a liquid formula to meet your nutritional needs. This formula contains all of the nutrients you need, just like a normal diet. There are many different types of formulas available today. Your doctor or dietitian will choose the formula to best meet your needs

Your Formula is ____

Tube Feeding Methods

Your medical team will determine the best method for your tube feeding and your schedule. The most common methods are:

Bolus Feedings
Gravity Feeding
Pump Feeding

You will be receiving _______________________________

Bolus Feeding Instructions

Supplies
- Formula (room temperature)
- Syringe (60 ml)
- Water (room temperature)

Preparation

1. Wash your hands thoroughly.
2. Wash and dry the top of the formula cans.
3. Shake the cans lightly.
4. Unclamp or uncap the feeding tube.
5. Sit or lie with your head at least 30 degrees upright and stay in this position for 30-60 minutes after feeding to prevent nausea or reflux.

Administration

1. Before you start the feeding, use the syringe to flush your feeding tube with _____ ml water.
2. Place the syringe tip into the feeding tube.
3. Remove the plunger from the barrel of the syringe and slowly pour the formula into the syringe. Allow the formula to drain into the tube with gravity OR use the plunger to push the formula into the tube.
4. After you've completed the feeding, flush the feeding tube with ___ ml of water.
5. Remove the syringe from the feeding tube and reclamp or recap the feeding tube.

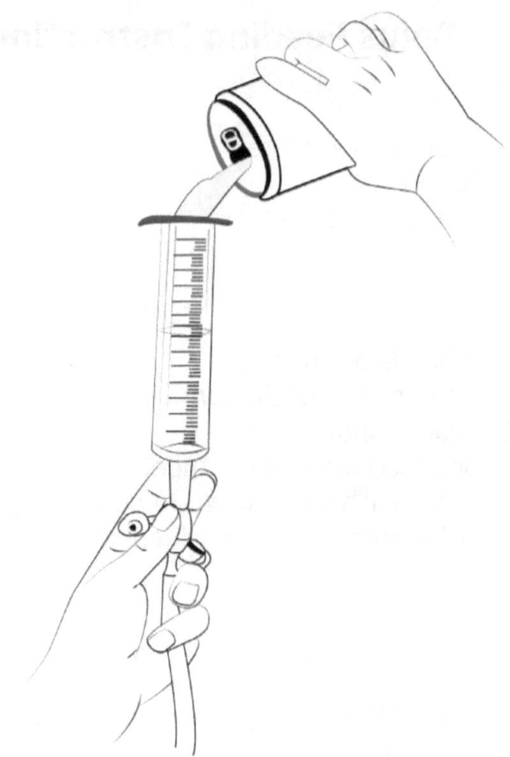

Tube Feeding Schedule

Feeding Method: ___________________________

Formula: ___________________________

Amount of Formula each day: ___________________________________

Feeding Schedule:

____

____

Flush feeding tube with _____ml water before and _____ml water after each feeding

Additional water: ___________________________

Gravity Feeding Instructions

Supplies
- Feeding container and tubing (gravity set)
- Formula (room temperature)
- Pole
- Syringe (60 ml)
- Water (room temperature)

Preparation

1. Wash hands thoroughly.
2. Wash and dry the top of the formula containers
3. Shake containers well
4. Pour the formula into the feeding container and close cap
5. Hand feeding container on a pole at least 18 inches above the stomach
6. Sit or lie at least 30 degrees upright and remain in this position for 30-60 minutes after each feeding to prevent reflux or nausea

Administration

1. Uncap or unclamp the feeding tube
2. Use the syringe to flush the feeding tube with _____ ml water
3. Connect the tip of the gravity set into the feeding tube
4. Open the flow regular clamp to adjust the flow rate. Tube feeds will begin
5. After feeding, close and disconnect the gravity set from the feeding tube
6. Use the syringe to flush the feeding tube with _____ ml water
7. Reclamp or recap the feeding tube

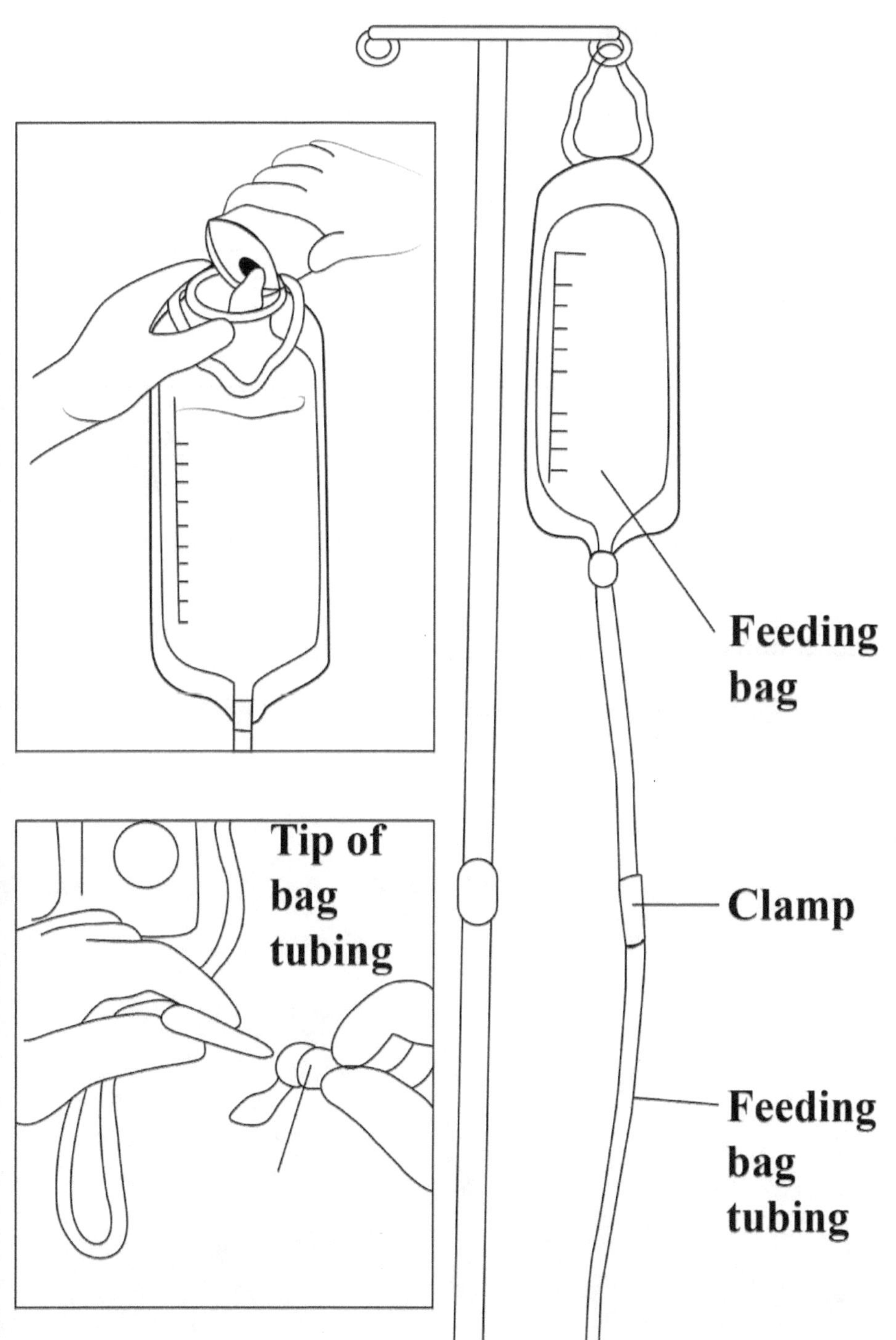

Tip of
bag
tubing
Feeding
bag
Clamp
Feeding
bag
tubing

Tube Feeding Schedule

Feeding Method:	_______________________

Formula:	____________________________

Amount of Formula each day:	________________________________

Feeding Schedule:

____

____

Flush feeding tube with _____ml water before and _____ml water after each feeding

Additional water:	___________________________________

Pump Assisted Instructions

Supplies
- Enteral feeding pump
- Feeding container and tubing (pump set)
- Formula (room temperature)
- Pole or stand
- Syringe (60 mL)
- Water (room temperature)

Preparation
1. Wash hands thoroughly.
2. Rinse the top of the formula container or opening or wipe with a clean sponge or paper towel.
3. Shake the formula container.
4. Pour the formula into the feeding container and close cap OR insert the pump set into the pre-filled feeding container.
5. Fill a feeding container with water (if needed)
6. Hang the feeding container and water container on a pole at least 18 inches above the stomach.

Administration
1. Sit or lie with your head elevated at least 30 degrees upright and stay in this position for 30-60 minutes after feeding to prevent nausea or reflux.
2. Unclamp or uncap the feeding tube
3. Use the syringe to flush the feeding tube with _____ mL water
4. Connect the tip of the pump set to the feeding tube
5. Set the flow rate on the pump to _____ mL per hour
6. Set the flow rate for water flushes on the pump to _____ mL per hour or as directed
7. If roller clamp present, open clamp on the pump set.
8. Start the pump.
9. Run for _____ hours
10. After feeding, disconnect the pump set and recap the end of the pump set
11. Use syringe to flush the feeding tube with _____ mL water
12. Reclamp or recap the feeding tube

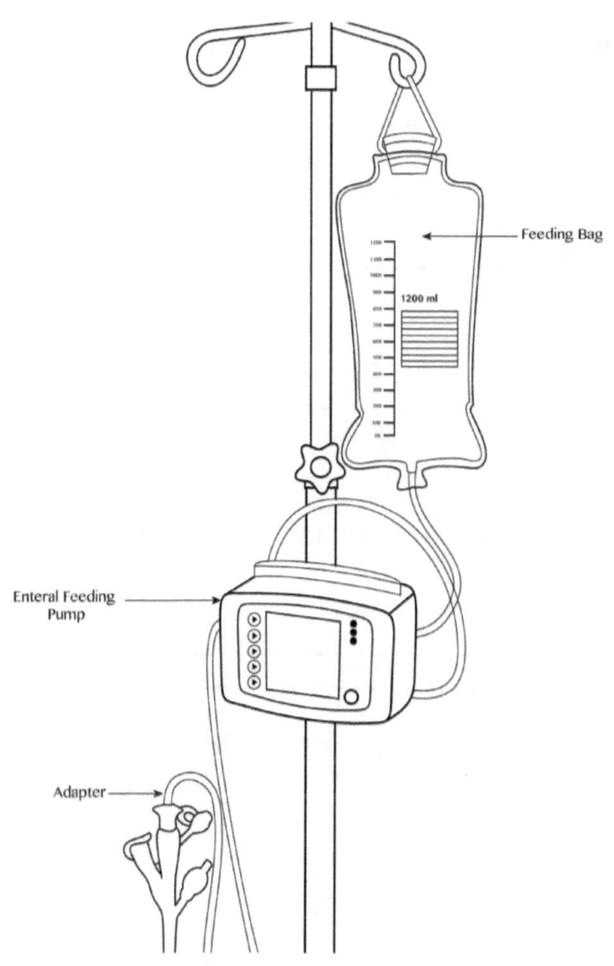

Feeding Bag
1200 ml
Enteral Feeding
Pump
Adapter

Tube Feeding Schedule

Feeding Method: _______________________

Formula: _______________________________

Amount of Formula each day: ___________________________________

Feeding Schedule:

____

____

Flush feeding tube with _____ml water before and _____ml water after each feeding

Additional water flushes: ___________________________________

Caring for the Feeding Tube Site

Gastrostomy or Jejunostomy

After you've had a tube inserted, keeping the skin around the tube site clean and dry is important to prevent infection and skin breakdown. You will need mild soap, gauze squares, and cotton swabs. Clean around the site daily or as recommended by your doctor

1. Fill a small container with soap and water. Wet gauze square and use to clean the skin around the tube. Start cleaning next to the tube and then work outwards to clear away any bacteria.
2. If the tube has a disk near the skin, use the cotton swab to clean under the disk. Avoid pulling the tube.
3. Use a second gauze square damp with water only to wipe away any soap residue.
4. Allow the area to dry.

Check the tube site every day for soreness, swelling, drainage, or other problems. Some mild drainage can occur. Clean any moisture from the area promptly and use a small dressing if desired. For any foul-smelling drainage or excessive drainage, contact your healthcare team promptly.

Storing Tube Feeding Formulas

It's important to store your formula properly. A tube feeding formula is food and can cause illness if not handled and stored as directed.

- Store any unopened cans or containers in a clean and dry place at room temperature. There is no need to store unopened formula in a refrigerator unless directed by the manufacturer.
- If only part of a container of formula is used, cover the container with plastic wrap and label it with the date and time it was opened. Store any opened formula in a refrigerator.
- Use any opened formula within 24 hours. Discard any unused formula past this time frame.
- If using a formula that has been refrigerated, remove and let sit at room temperature 30 minutes before using to avoid any stomach discomfort. Leave it covered until ready for use.
- Do not heat formula in a microwave or on a stovetop.

Administering Medications

After you have a feeding tube placed, many or all of your medications will be administered through this tube. Follow your healthcare professional's directions for taking medication. Liquid medications are the best choice when available. Any pills should be crushed into a fine powder and dissolved in water to administer through your tube.

Ask your nurse, doctor, or pharmacist for instructions on:

- How to crush medications
- How much water to mix with medication and water flushes with medications
- Which medications can or cannot be crushed
- Any other information to know when giving medications through a feeding tube

Your pharmacist or doctor may provide specific directions which should be followed. Many medications can be delivered using these instructions

Instructions

1. Unclamp or uncap the feeding tube.
2. Use a 60 mL syringe to flush the feeding tube with 15-30 mL warm water or as directed by your healthcare professional.
3. Using a 60 mL syringe, draw up the correct dose of liquid medication or crushed medication mixed with water.
4. Connect the syringe into the feeding tube.
5. Gentle press the plunger to push the water and medication into the tube.
6. Remove the syringe from the feeding tube and refill syringe with 15-30 mL warm water. Flush the water through the tube. You may need additional water flushes to flush all the medication from the syringe.
7. Reclamp or reclose the feeding tube.

Adjusting to Tube Feeding

It may be difficult to change from eating to tube feeding. Many people miss their favorite foods or the ability to enjoy a family meal. You can use these strategies to adjust to this change:

- Take your feedings at the same time as the rest of the family eats. If you have to take your feedings at other times, sit with family and friends at mealtimes to socialize and then follow your tube feeding schedule between meals.
- Use mouthwashes and lip balms to freshen your mouth. Follow the oral hygiene recommended by your doctor

Troubleshooting

Although tube feeds are standard today, you may experience some problems or challenges at home. These are the most common complications seen with tube feeds and most common solutions. When in doubt, be sure to contact your healthcare team.

Clogging

All tubes have the risk of clogging which may be due to the following causes:
- Inadequate water flushes
- Not flushing between medications
- High-fiber or concentrated tube feeding formula

Solutions:

- Follow the water flush recommendations given by your medical team. Water is the preferred fluid to use for flushes and avoid sodas or juices through the tube as they may cause breakdown of the tube.
- Crush medications and use liquid forms of medications when available
- Give medications separately with water flushes between each medication
- Unclog the tube
  - Check that the tube is not kinked
  - If you can see the blocked area, try lightly massaging the area to remove the blockage. Run your thumb and forefinger down the tube lightly, applying mild pressure.
  - If still clogged, insert a syringe into the end of the tube. Pull back the plunger to remove as much fluid as possible. Discard the fluid
  - Insert the syringe with ~10 ml warm water into the tube and move the plunger back and forth.
  - If the tube is still not clear, clamp for 5-15 minutes, letting the warm water stay in the tube.
  - Fill the syringe with ~10 ml warm water and try again. Repeat several times until the tube is unclogged.
  - If the tube remains clogged, report to urgent care

Stomach Pain/Discomfort

If you feel nausea, bloating, gas pain, belching, or heartburn, consider changing your tube feeding schedule. Common reasons can include:

- Too much volume at one time
- Giving feeds to closely together

Solutions:

- Give your tube feeding slowly. Don't force the feeding. If you start to feel full, wait an hour before trying again.
- Don't give yourself a feeding if you feel stomach pain or if you vomit
- Sit upright during feeds and at least one hour afterwards
- If nausea continues, hold the feeding for a few hours. Call your doctor if you're nauseated more than 24 hours.

Diarrhea

Since tube feeding formulas are liquid, your stools will likely be soft instead of formed. This is normal and not a cause for concern. However, if you experience watery stools with 6-8 or more bowel movements a day, then you are experiencing diarrhea. Common reasons can include:

- Spoiled formula or poor handwashing
- Intolerance of tube feeding formula
- Intolerance of tube feeding regimen
- Other digestive problem/illness

Solutions:

- If you are pump-assisted tube feeds, slow down the rate. Call your dietitian to determine how to adjust your feeding.
- If you are on bolus tube feeds, slow down the rate of the tube feeding. Divide the feedings into smaller amounts and take them more often. For example, if you take 480 mL of formula three times a day, you can change to 240 mL six times a day.
- Ensure that you are following proper handwashing recommendations. Discard formula that has been open more than

48 hours, refrigerate opened cans, and never use any formula past
its expiration date.
- If diarrhea continues for more than 48-72 hours, call your doctor.

Constipation

Most tube feedings are low in fiber and you may have bowel movements
every one or two days. If you have not had bowel movements in two days
or you're experiencing hard stools, you are constipated.

Solutions:

- Increase your physical activity, if possible
- Increase your tube feeding water flushes, if not on a fluid
  restriction
- Call your doctor if you have not had a bowel movement in 3-4 days

Vomiting or Aspiration

Vomiting is a dangerous problem that you may experience with tube feeds.
You may also have vomit or saliva inhaled into your lungs which is known
as aspiration. This usually occurs when you vomit and then cannot clear
your throat of these fluids. This is a serious complication and can cause
problems. Potential reasons for vomiting or aspiration include:

- Intolerance of your tube feeding formula or rate
- Giving yourself a feeding while laying down

Solutions

- Give yourself the tube feeding formula as directed. Do not increase
  the rate or volume of the feeds unless directed by your doctor or
  dietitian.
- Do not give yourself feeds of unapproved formulas or liquids
  through your tube
- Slow down your rate of feeds or give yourself a smaller volume with
  each feed
- Keep your head up 30-45 degrees when you give yourself feeds
  and for at least 30 minutes after feeds.
- If you are choking or having difficulty breathing, stop the feeds
  right away and call your doctor or an ambulance

Dehydration

Your doctor or dietitian will provide you with a tube feeding regimen that will include water flushes when you leave the hospital. You should follow this regimen but your fluid needs may change over time. Common reasons for dehydration include:

- Fluid losses- diarrhea or excessive sweating
- Inadequate water flushes

Solutions:

- Make sure that you're giving yourself both the formula and the water flushes each day (see your Tube Feeding Prescription).
- If you tend to sweat a lot, have a fever, or are having diarrhea, increase your water flushes. Check with your doctor or dietitian to determine how much to increase your water flushes before making any changes

Tube Removal

There is a possibility that your tube can fall out or become misplaced. This can cause medical complications if the tube is not located properly.

Solution:

- Go immediately to the closest emergency room to have the tube replaced. Bring the tube with you and have the contact information for your doctor available, if possible.

Mouth Dryness

If you aren't able to eat or drink anything, you may notice that you have bad breath or mouth dryness.

Solutions:

- Brush your mouth at least twice a day
- Rinse your mouth with a mouthwash or a mild salt or baking soda solution (1 tsp salt or baking soda in a glass of water). Repeat several times a day

- If allowed, chew sugarless gum or sugarless candy
- Use a lip balm for dry lips

If you experience bleeding in your mouth area, sores or other areas of irritation, check with your health care professional for instructions.

Missed Feedings

There will be times that you miss your feeding or start feedings late. This is usually not a serious problem unless you have diabetes or you are missing feedings on a regular basis.

Solutions:

- For pump-assisted feedings, adjust your rate to get in the amount that you need. You can also run the pump for a longer period of time to make up for the time that you missed.
    - Instead of 60 ml/hr over 10 hours, increase the rate to run 75 ml/hr for 8 hours. Both regimens will provide same 600 ml volume.
    - If your tube feed runs from 10 PM-6 AM, you can run it from 12 AM-8 AM
    - Check with your dietitian or doctor for any adjustments as you may not be able to change your schedule
- For bolus feeds, add a missed feed onto the end of your day. If you miss your first feed at 8 AM, add a missed feed in the evening.
- If you don't have time to catch up on your feeds, don't worry about one day where you didn't get adequate nutrition. However, if you can't keep up with your feeds for 2-3 days of the week, talk to your doctor or dietitian about adjusting your schedule.

Other Problems

You may experience other problems or concerns related to your tube feedings. If you run into any problems or concerns not listed here, contact your healthcare professional:

____

____

Finding Support

Many people feel overwhelmed with their feeding tube. The transition to home tube feeds can be a challenge and you're not alone. Whether you are a person with tube feeds or a caregiver, you can benefit from having community and resources. Your first resource for any problems should be your doctor or dietitian who is familiar with your health.

For additional resources, these are some of the best places to find support and guidance in addition to your healthcare professionals. The content on these websites is for educational purposes and should NOT be considered medical advice. It should not replace the advice of your healthcare team. Please consult with your healthcare professional and team regarding any questions about your home tube feeding plan.

The Oley Foundation

The Oley Foundation is a national non-profit organization that provides education, information, and support to individuals on tube feeds.
www.oley.org

CaringBridge

CaringBridge provides websites that connect people who are experiencing health problems to family and friends.
www.caringbridge.org

Tube Feeding Awareness

This website is a community of parents who are raising children with feeding tubes who want to share their experiences in addition to raising awareness or tube feeding.
www.feedingtubeawareness.com

MIC-KEY Tube

This brand of feeding tubes is designed to help individuals and caregivers share and learn more about feeding tubes and care. They provide online tools and resources to manage tube feeds.
www.mic-key.com

A.S.P.E.N.

The American Society for Parenteral and Enteral Nutrition (ASPEN) is an organization dedicated to improving patient care by researching nutrition support and providing guidelines on best practices.
www.nutritioncare.org

Definitions

Aspiration: Fluid inhaled into your lungs. This is life-threatening

Bolus tube feeds: A method for giving a certain volume of feeds several times a day

Constipation: Not having a bowel movement for more than two days or experiencing hard stools

Continuous tube feeds: A constant method for giving feedings over 8-24 hours

Dehydration: receiving less water than your body needs

Diarrhea: Watery stools and more than 6-8 bowel movements a day

Feeding tube: A plastic tube that allows formula to pass into the stomach or intestine for nutrition or medications

Feeding Pump: a machine that's used to control the flow of a tube feeding formula

Formula: A liquid nutrition product designed to be a sole source of nutrition

Gravity Feeding: A feeding method in which a formula drips down through a feeding tube from a container placed above your stomach

Jejunostomy Tube (J-tube): A feeding tube that ends in the small intestine

Jejunum: The second part of the small intestine

Gastrostomy Tube (PEG or G-tube): A tube that ends in the stomach

Pump Feeding: A feeding method that uses a pump to move formula through the feeding tube

Stoma: Opening in the abdominal wall through a g-tube or j-tube enters the body

Syringe: A hollow, plastic tube with a plunger used to draw fluid from or inject fluid into a feeding tube

Syringe feeding: A feeding method in which formula flows from a syringe into the feeding tube or is injected into the feeding tube with a syringe

Units of Measure:
- 30 milliliters (mL) = 1 ounce (oz.)
- 240 mL = 8 ounces = 1 standard measuring cup

Tube Feeding Journal

Date	Sun	Mon	Tues	Wed	Thurs	Fri	Sat
Weight (Lbs)							
Amount of Formula (mL)							
Amount of Water (mL)							
Other fluids put through tube (description and mL)							
Number of stools and consistency (hard, soft, watery)							
Other							

References

Charney P, Malone A. ADA Pocket Guide to Enteral Nutrition. American Dietetic Associati; 2006.

Ed. CM. The A.S.P.E.N. Adult Nutrition Support Core Curriculum. American Society for Parenteral & Enteral Nutrition; 2012.

Feeding Tube Awareness Foundation. Feeding Tube Awareness Foundation. http://www.feedingtubeawareness.org/. Accessed March 5, 2018.

Oley Foundation. Oley Foundation. http://oley.org/. Accessed March 5, 2018.

www.ingramcontent.com/pod-product-compliance
Lightning Source LLC
Chambersburg PA
CBHW021149260726
48656CB00025B/2327